Anatomy of Liver

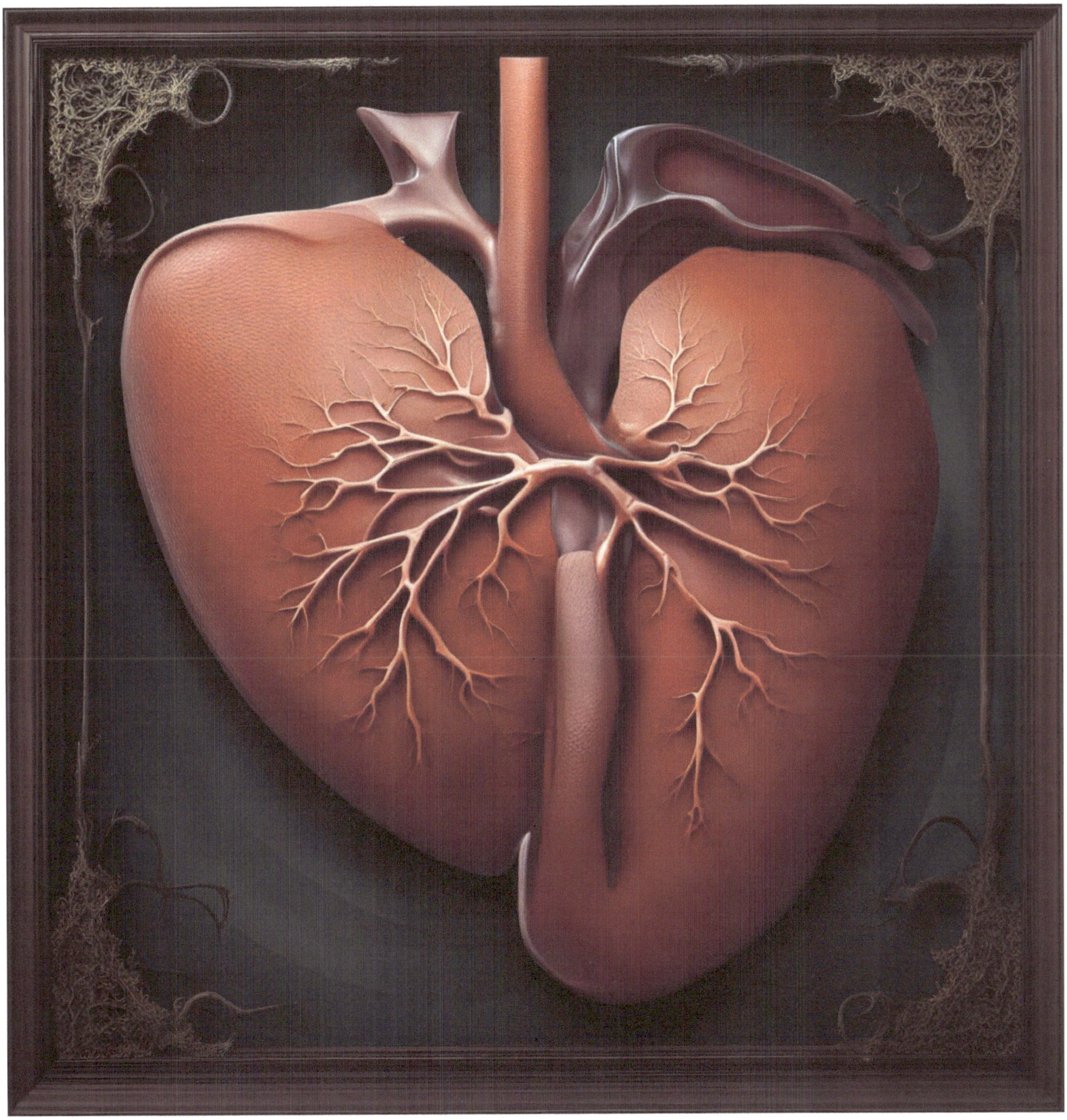

I'd be happy to provide you with an overview of the anatomy of the human liver. However, writing an entire ebook would be a lengthy process. Instead, I can give you a brief summary of the key points to get you started. If you have specific questions or need more detailed information on a particular aspect, feel free to ask!

I would like to express my heartfelt gratitude to my mom to make this ebook

Thanks a lot!

[Anatomy of human liver]

By

Dr. Suriya prakash R

Department of general medicine

Title: "The Comprehensive Guide to the Anatomy of the Human Liver"

Chapter 1: Introduction
- Features of liver
- Importance of the liver

Chapter 2: Overview of the Liver
- Location and size
- Functions of the liver
- Importance in metabolism

Chapter 3: External Anatomy
- Lobes of the liver
- Blood supply and vascular anatomy
- Biliary system

Chapter 4: Internal Anatomy
- Hepatic cells and their arrangement
- Sinusoids and hepatic plates
- Functional units of the liver

Chapter 5: Microscopic Anatomy
- Hepatocytes and their functions

- Kupffer cells and their role
- Liver sinusoidal endothelial cells

Chapter 6: Blood Supply
- Portal vein and hepatic artery
- Hepatic portal system
- The liver sinusoids
- Hepatic veins

Chapter 7: Biliary System
- Structure of bile ducts
- Gallbladder and its function
- Bile production and transport

Chapter 8: Liver Functions
- Metabolism of Nutrients
- Detoxification and Toxin Removal
- Storage of Vitamins and Minerals
- Synthesis of Proteins, Including Clotting Factors

Chapter 9: Innervation
- Nerves and ganglia
- Autonomic control of liver functions
- Role in digestion and metabolism

Chapter 10: Liver Development
- Embryological development of the liver
- Changes throughout life

Chapter 11: Common Liver Conditions
- Hepatitis
- Cirrhosis
- Liver cancer
- Liver abscess
- Fatty liver disease

Chapter 12: Diagnostic Techniques
- Imaging methods
- Blood tests
- Biopsy

Chapter 13: Surgical Anatomy
- Liver resection
- Transplantation
- Surgical considerations

Chapter 14: Maintaining Liver Health
- Healthy lifestyle choices
- Diet and nutrition
- Liver detoxification myths

Chapter 1: Introduction

Features of liver

The liver is a large and solid gland situated in the right upper quadrant of the abdominal cavity. In the living subject, the liver is reddish brown in colour, soft in consistency, and very friable. It weighs about 1600 g in males and about 1300 g in females.

Importance of the liver

The liver is a vital organ responsible for numerous crucial functions in the body, including metabolism, detoxification, storage of nutrients, and synthesis of essential proteins. Its importance lies in maintaining overall health and homeostasis, as dysfunction can lead to severe medical conditions, making it imperative to care for and protect the liver throughout life.

Chapter 2: Overview of the Liver

Location and size

The liver occupies the whole of the right hypochondrium, the greater part of the epigastrium, and extends into the left hypochondrium reaching up to the left lateral line. From the above, it will be obvious that most of the liver is covered by ribs and costal cartilages, except in the upper part of the epigastrium where it is in contact with the anterior abdominal wall. The liver is the largest gland in the body. It secretes bile and performs various other metabolic functions. The liver is also called the 'hepar' from which we have the adjective 'hepatic' applied to many structures connected with the organ.

The average size of the human liver is approximately 6.5 to 7.5 inches (16.5 to 19 centimeters) in length and 4.5 to 5.5 inches (11.4 to 14 centimeters) in width. It's about the size of a football and typically weighs around 3 pounds (1.36 kilograms) in a healthy adult. However, liver size can vary among individuals, and it can change due to factors such as age, health, and body composition.

Functions of the liver

Liver is a dual organ having both secretory and excretory functions.

Liver is an indispensable gland of the body.

- Metabolism of carbohydrates, fats and proteins
- Synthesis of bile and prothrombin
- Excretion of drugs, toxins, poisons, cholesterol, bile pigments and heavy metals
- Protective by conjugation, destruction, phagocytosis, antibody formation and excretion
- Storage of glycogen, iron, fat, vitamins A and D.

Hepatic Lobes Liver is made up of many lobes called hepatic lobes. Each lobe consists of many lobules called hepatic lobules.

Hepatic Lobules Hepatic lobule is the structural and functional unit of liver. There are about 50,000 to 100,000 lobules in the liver. The lobule is a honeycomb-like structure and it is made up of liver cells called hepatocytes.

Portal Triads Each lobule is surrounded by many portal triads. Each portal triad consists of three vessels:

1. A branch of hepatic artery

2. A branch of portal vein

3. A tributary of bile duct.

Branches of hepatic artery and portal vein open into the sinusoid. Sinusoid opens into the central vein. Central vein empties into hepatic vein. Bile is secreted by hepatic cells and emptied into bile canaliculus. From canaliculus, the bile enters the tributary of bile duct. Tributaries of bile duct from canaliculi of neighboring lobules unite to form small bile ducts. These small bile ducts join together and finally form left and right hepatic ducts, which emerge out of liver.

Importance in metabolism

The liver plays a crucial role in metabolism, making it one of the most important organs in the body for maintaining overall health. Here are some key aspects of the liver's role in metabolism:

Carbohydrate Metabolism: The liver helps regulate blood sugar levels by storing excess glucose as glycogen and releasing it when needed. It also converts non-carbohydrate sources (like amino acids and glycerol) into glucose through a process called gluconeogenesis.

Fat Metabolism: The liver is involved in the synthesis of lipids (fats) and the breakdown of fatty acids for energy production. It also produces bile, which is essential for the digestion and absorption of fats.

Protein Metabolism: It synthesizes and breaks down proteins, ensuring a balance of amino acids in the bloodstream. The liver also removes excess ammonia, a toxic byproduct of protein metabolism, by converting it into urea for excretion.

Detoxification: The liver plays a crucial role in detoxifying the body by processing and neutralizing toxins, drugs, and metabolic waste products. It converts harmful substances into water-soluble compounds that can be excreted by the kidneys.

Storage: The liver stores essential nutrients like vitamins (A, D, B12), minerals (iron), and glycogen. These reserves can be mobilized when the body requires them.

Metabolic Regulation: The liver is involved in regulating various metabolic processes, such as hormone metabolism, cholesterol synthesis, and the conversion of vitamin D into its active form.

Immune Function: It participates in the body's immune response by filtering and removing bacteria and foreign particles from the bloodstream.

In summary, the liver's role in metabolism is multifaceted, and it is essential for maintaining a stable internal environment and overall metabolic health in the body. Dysfunction of the liver can lead to various metabolic disorders and health issues.

Chapter 3: External Anatomy

External Features

The liver is wedge-shaped. It resembles a four-sided pyramid laid on one side Surfaces It has five surfaces. These are:

1 Anterior,

2 Posterior,

3 Superior,

4 Inferior, and

5 Right.

Out of these, the inferior surface is well defined because it is demarcated, anteriorly, by a sharp inferior border. The other surfaces are more or less continuous with each other and are imperfectly separated from one another by ill-defined, rounded borders.

Prominent Border The inferior border is sharp anteriorly where it separates the anterior surface from the inferior surface. It is somewhat rounded laterally where it separates the right surface from the inferior surface. The sharp anterior part is marked by:

a. An interlobar notch or the notch for the ligamentum teres.

b. A cystic notch for the fundus of the gallbladder.

In the epigastrium, the inferior border extends from the left 8th costal cartilage to the right 9th costal cartilage.

Lobes of the liver

The liver is divided into right and left lobes by the attachment of the falciform ligament anteriorly and superiorly; by the fissure for the ligamentum teres inferiorly; and by the fissure for the ligamentum venosum posteriorly.

The right lobe is much larger than the left lobe, and forms five-sixths of the liver. It contributes to all the five surfaces of the liver, and presents the caudate and quadrate lobes.

The caudate lobe is situated on the posterior surface. It is bounded on the right by the groove for the inferior vena cava, on the left by the fissure for the ligamentum venosum, and inferiorly by the porta hepatis. Above, it is continuous with the superior surface. Below and to the right, just behind the porta hepatis, it is connected to the right lobe of the liver by the caudate process. Below and to the left, it presents a small rounded elevation called the papillary process.

The quadrate lobe is situated on the inferior surface, and is rectangular in shape. It is bounded anteriorly by the inferior border, posteriorly by the porta hepatis, on the right by the fossa for the gallbladder, and on the left by the fissure for the ligamentum teres.

The porta hepatis is a deep, transverse fissure about 5 cm long, situated on the inferior surface of the right lobe of the liver. It lies between the caudate lobe above and the quadrate lobe below and in front. The portal vein, the hepatic artery and the hepatic plexus of nerves enter the liver through the porta hepatis, while the right and left hepatic ducts and a few lymphatics leave it. The relations within; the porta hepatis are from behind forwards are the portal vein, the hepatic artery and the hepatic ducts. The lips of the porta hepatis provide attachment to the lesser omentum.

The left lobe of the liver is much smaller than the right lobe and forms only one-sixth of the liver. It is flattened from above downwards. Near the fissure for the ligamentum venosum, its inferior surface presents a rounded elevation, called the omental tuberosity or tuber omentale.

Blood supply and vascular anatomy

Arterial Supply The liver receives 20% of its blood supply through the hepatic artery, and 80% through the portal vein. Before entering the liver, both the hepatic artery and the portal vein divide into right and left branches. Within the liver, they redivide to form segmental vessels which further divide to form interlobular vessels which run in the portal canals. Further ramifications of the interlobular branches open into the hepatic sinusoids. Thus the hepatic arterial blood mixes with the portal venous blood in the sinusoids. There are no anastomoses between adjoining hepatic arterial territories and hence each branch is an end artery.

Venous Drainage Hepatic sinusoids drain into interlobular veins, which join to form sublobular veins. These in turn unite to form the hepatic veins which drain directly into the inferior vena cava. These veins provide great support to the liver, besides the intra-abdominal pressure.

The hepatic veins are arranged in two groups: upper and lower. The upper group consists of three large veins: Right, left and middle, which emerge through the upper part of the groove for the inferior vena cava, and open directly into the vena cava. These veins keep the liver suspended. The lower group consists of a variable number of small veins from the right lobe and the caudate lobe which emerge through the lower part of the caval groove and open into the vena cava.

Microscopically, the tributaries of hepatic veins, i.e. central veins are seen as separate channels from those of the portal radicles.

Lymphatic Drainage The superficial lymphatics of the liver run on the surface of the organ beneath the peritoneum, and terminate in caval, hepatic, paracardial and coeliac lymph nodes. Some vessels from the coronary ligament may directly join the thoracic duct.

The deep lymphatics end partly in the nodes around the end of the inferior vena cava, and partly in the hepatic nodes.

Biliary system

Biliary system or extrahepatic biliary apparatus is formed by gallbladder and extrahepatic bile ducts (bile ducts outside the liver). Right and left hepatic bile ducts which come out of liver join to form common hepatic duct. It unites with the cystic duct from gallbladder to form common bile duct. All these ducts have similar structures. Common bile duct unites with pancreatic duct to form the common hepatopancreatic duct or ampulla of Vater, which opens into the duodenum. There is a sphincter called sphincter of Oddi at the lower part of common bile duct, before it joins the pancreatic duct. It is formed by smooth muscle fibers of common bile duct. It is commonly kept closed, so the bile secreted from liver enters gallbladder where it is stored. Upon appropriate stimulation, the sphincter opens and allows flow of bile from gallbladder into the intestine.

Chapter 4: Internal Anatomy

The internal anatomy of the liver includes two main lobes (right and left), microscopic lobules containing hepatocytes, bile ducts for bile transport, a dual blood supply from the hepatic artery and portal vein, sinusoids for nutrient exchange, Kupffer cells for immune function, the gallbladder for bile storage, the hepatic portal system for nutrient processing, and connective tissue for support. These structures collectively enable the liver to perform its vital metabolic and detoxification functions.

Hepatic cells and their arrangement

Hepatic cells, also known as hepatocytes, are the primary functional cells of the liver. They are arranged in a specific pattern within liver lobules to facilitate their various metabolic functions. Here's an overview of hepatic cells and their arrangement:

Hepatocytes: Hepatocytes are the main cell type in the liver, making up about 70-80% of the liver's mass. They perform a wide range of metabolic functions, including the synthesis of proteins, lipids, and carbohydrates, detoxification of harmful substances, and storage of nutrients.

Arrangement in Lobules: Hepatocytes are arranged in a hexagonal pattern within liver lobules, which are the structural and functional units of the liver. This arrangement allows for efficient exchange of substances between hepatocytes and the blood in sinusoids.

Central Vein: Each liver lobule has a central vein at its center. The sinusoids converge toward the central vein, and blood flows out of the lobule through this central vein.

Zonation: Hepatocytes are not uniform throughout the lobule. There is a zonation pattern, meaning that different regions of the lobule have specialized functions. For example, hepatocytes closer to the portal triads are more involved in nutrient processing, while those near the central vein are focused on detoxification and waste removal.

The arrangement of hepatocytes in hexagonal lobules, along with the unique structure of sinusoids and the presence of portal triads, optimizes the liver's efficiency in processing and regulating nutrients, detoxifying the blood, and performing its essential metabolic functions.

Sinusoids and hepatic plates

Sinusoids: Sinusoids are specialized capillaries located between rows of hepatocytes in the liver lobules. They have a unique structure with a discontinuous endothelial lining, which facilitates the exchange of nutrients, oxygen, and waste products between blood and hepatocytes.

Hepatic Plates Hepatocytes are arranged in columns, which form the hepatic plates. Each plate is made up of two columns of cells. In between the two columns of each plate lies a bile canaliculus. In between the neighboring plates, a blood space called sinusoid is present. Sinusoid is lined by the endothelial cells. In between the endothelial cells some special macrophages called Kupffer cells are present.

Functional units of the liver

The functional unit of the liver is the "liver lobule." Liver lobules are hexagonal structures composed of hepatocytes (liver cells) arranged around a central vein. They are the basic building blocks of the liver and facilitate various metabolic functions, including nutrient processing, detoxification, and bile production. Blood flows through sinusoids within the lobule, allowing hepatocytes to perform their tasks and maintain overall liver function.

Chapter 5: Microscopic Anatomy

The microscopic anatomy of the liver reveals a complex structure comprising liver lobules, hepatocytes (liver cells), sinusoids (specialized blood vessels), and portal triads (containing hepatic portal vein, hepatic artery, and bile duct). Liver lobules are hexagonal units where hepatocytes process nutrients, detoxify the blood, and produce bile. Sinusoids allow for nutrient exchange, while portal triads supply blood and bile. This intricate arrangement optimizes the liver's metabolic functions, making it a vital organ for digestion and detoxification.

Hepatocytes and their functions

Hepatocytes are the primary functional cells of the liver, and they perform a wide range of vital functions essential for maintaining overall health. Here are some of the key functions of hepatocytes:

Metabolism of Nutrients: Hepatocytes play a central role in the metabolism of carbohydrates, lipids, and proteins. They store excess glucose as glycogen and release it when needed to regulate blood sugar levels. They also synthesize and break down fats and proteins.

Detoxification: Hepatocytes are responsible for detoxifying the blood by processing and neutralizing various toxins, drugs, and metabolic waste products. They convert harmful substances into water-soluble compounds that can be excreted from the body.

Bile Production: Hepatocytes produce bile, a greenish-yellow fluid that is essential for digestion. Bile is stored in the gallbladder and released into the small intestine to emulsify fats and aid in their absorption.

Synthesis of Proteins: The liver produces a variety of proteins, including blood clotting factors, albumin (which helps maintain blood volume and pressure), and enzymes necessary for digestion.

Regulation of Cholesterol Levels: Hepatocytes play a role in regulating cholesterol levels in the body by producing and secreting cholesterol and other lipoproteins.

Metabolism of Drugs and Hormones: They metabolize drugs and hormones, helping to regulate their levels in the bloodstream.

Storage of Glycogen: Hepatocytes store glycogen, which can be converted back into glucose when the body needs an energy boost.

Immune Functions: These cells have immune-related functions and can remove bacteria, toxins, and other foreign substances from the bloodstream.

Synthesis of Blood Proteins: Hepatocytes produce essential blood proteins, including clotting factors and complement proteins involved in the immune response.

In summary, hepatocytes are versatile cells responsible for numerous metabolic, detoxification, and regulatory functions in the liver. Their role in processing nutrients, detoxifying the body, and maintaining metabolic balance makes them critical for overall health and well-being.

Kupffer cells and their role

Kupffer cells are specialized macrophages found in the liver, specifically within the sinusoids, which are the specialized capillaries that run between hepatocytes (liver cells). These cells play a crucial role in the liver's overall function and immune defense. Here's an overview of Kupffer cells and their role:

Phagocytosis: Kupffer cells are primarily known for their ability to phagocytose (engulf and digest) foreign particles, such as bacteria, viruses, toxins, and worn-out blood cells, that enter the liver through the bloodstream. This function helps to maintain a clean and sterile environment within the liver.

Detoxification: Kupffer cells contribute to the liver's detoxification processes by capturing and breaking down harmful substances that might enter the liver through the portal vein, helping to prevent these toxins from reaching systemic circulation.

Immune Response: These cells are integral to the liver's immune response. When Kupffer cells detect pathogens or foreign particles, they can trigger an immune response by releasing cytokines and other signaling molecules. This response can activate other immune cells in the liver and contribute to the overall immune defense of the body.

Iron Recycling: Kupffer cells also play a role in recycling iron from old red blood cells. They capture and break down these cells, releasing iron for reuse in the body.

Inflammation Regulation: Kupffer cells can modulate inflammation in the liver. While they can contribute to inflammation when necessary to combat infection, they also help regulate the resolution of inflammation to prevent excessive damage to liver tissue.

Tissue Repair: In addition to their immune functions, Kupffer cells can be involved in tissue repair and regeneration within the liver, particularly after injury or infection.

In summary, Kupffer cells are resident macrophages in the liver that act as a frontline defense against pathogens and toxins entering the bloodstream from the digestive tract. Their role in phagocytosis, detoxification, immune response, and iron recycling makes them essential for maintaining the liver's health and function.

Liver sinusoidal endothelial cells

Liver sinusoidal endothelial cells (LSECs) are specialized endothelial cells that line the sinusoids within the liver. Sinusoids are the unique capillaries found in the liver, situated between rows of hepatocytes (liver cells). LSECs play a crucial role in maintaining the liver's structure and function. Here's an overview of liver sinusoidal endothelial cells and their functions:

Fenestrations: LSECs have small pores or fenestrations in their cytoplasmic membrane. These fenestrations allow for the exchange of substances between the blood in the sinusoids and hepatocytes, enabling the efficient passage of nutrients, oxygen, and waste products.

Blood Filtration: LSECs act as a filter for blood entering the liver. They can capture and remove particles, such as bacteria, toxins, and worn-out blood cells, from the bloodstream, helping to maintain a clean and sterile environment within the liver.

Endocytosis: LSECs are involved in the endocytosis of various substances from the blood, including lipoproteins and hormones. They can regulate the levels of these substances in the liver, affecting metabolic processes.

Immune Functions: Liver sinusoidal endothelial cells play a role in the liver's immune response. They can interact with immune cells, such as Kupffer cells (resident macrophages) and lymphocytes, to initiate and regulate immune reactions in response to infections or injuries.

Angiocrine Functions: LSECs secrete angiocrine factors, which are signaling molecules that help regulate angiogenesis (the formation of new blood vessels) and tissue regeneration within the liver. This function is essential for liver repair and regeneration after injury.

Liver Fibrosis: LSECs are involved in liver fibrosis, a process that occurs in chronic liver diseases. Their dysfunction can contribute to fibrosis by promoting the buildup of scar tissue within the liver.

Regulation of Blood Flow: LSECs play a role in regulating blood flow within the liver by releasing factors that influence the constriction or dilation of blood vessels.

In summary, liver sinusoidal endothelial cells are a specialized type of endothelial cell uniquely adapted to the liver's sinusoidal environment. Their functions in fenestration, filtration, endocytosis, immune response, angiogenesis regulation, and blood flow make them integral to the liver's metabolic, detoxification, and immune functions.

Chapter 6: Blood Supply

Portal vein and hepatic artery

The portal vein and hepatic artery are two distinct blood vessels that provide the liver with its dual blood supply, each carrying blood with different characteristics and functions:

Portal Vein:

Origin: The portal vein originates from various branches of veins in the digestive organs, including the stomach, small intestine, and large intestine.

Blood Composition: The blood in the portal vein is rich in nutrients absorbed from the digestive tract, such as glucose, amino acids, vitamins, and toxins. It is also relatively low in oxygen.

Function: The portal vein carries blood containing the products of digestion to the liver for processing. These nutrients are then metabolized, stored, or released into the bloodstream as needed. The liver detoxifies the blood by removing harmful substances.

Hepatic Artery:

Origin: The hepatic artery arises from the celiac trunk, which is a branch of the abdominal aorta.

Blood Composition: The blood in the hepatic artery is oxygen-rich and carries nutrients necessary for the liver's metabolic functions. It is also relatively low in nutrients like glucose, as it primarily supplies oxygen.

Function: The hepatic artery supplies oxygenated blood to the liver to meet its metabolic needs. Oxygen is essential for the liver to perform its various functions, including the synthesis of proteins, lipids, and the detoxification of blood.

In the liver, these two blood supplies merge within the sinusoids, specialized capillaries that run between hepatocytes (liver cells). This arrangement allows the liver to process and regulate the levels of nutrients, oxygen, and toxins in the blood, ensuring proper metabolic function and detoxification. The dual blood supply is a critical feature that makes the liver a central organ for metabolic and detoxification processes in the body.

Hepatic portal system

The hepatic portal system is a unique circulatory network that transports blood from the digestive organs to the liver before it enters the systemic circulation. It consists of the following key components:

Portal Vein: Blood from the stomach, small intestine, large intestine, and other digestive organs is collected into small veins, which then merge to form the portal vein. This vein carries nutrient-rich but oxygen-depleted blood to the liver.

Hepatic Portal Vein: The portal vein branches within the liver into smaller vessels, known as hepatic portal veins. These veins distribute the blood to various regions of the liver, ensuring that the liver has access to the products of digestion.

Liver Processing: Inside the liver, blood from the hepatic portal system comes into contact with hepatocytes (liver cells) and liver sinusoids. The hepatocytes process nutrients, detoxify harmful substances, and regulate blood sugar levels.

Detoxification: One crucial function of the hepatic portal system is detoxification. The liver filters and removes toxins, drugs, and other harmful substances from the blood before it enters the systemic circulation. This detoxification process is essential for maintaining overall health.

Metabolism and Nutrient Regulation: The liver also metabolizes nutrients absorbed from the digestive tract, storing, releasing, or converting them as needed to maintain a balanced internal environment. For example, it stores excess glucose as glycogen and releases it when blood sugar levels drop.

Bile Production: The liver produces bile, which is necessary for digestion. Bile is transported through the bile ducts to the gallbladder, where it is stored until it is released into the small intestine to aid in fat digestion.

Overall, the hepatic portal system allows the liver to act as a central processing unit for the nutrients and toxins absorbed from the digestive organs. This unique circulatory arrangement ensures that these substances are effectively metabolized, regulated, and detoxified before they enter the rest of the body's circulation.

The liver sinusoids

Liver sinusoids are specialized capillaries found within the liver, and they are a crucial component of the liver's unique structure and function. Here are key characteristics and functions of liver sinusoids:

Location: Liver sinusoids are located between rows of hepatocytes (liver cells) within liver lobules, which are the structural and functional units of the liver.

Structure: They have a unique and specialized structure. The endothelial cells lining the sinusoids have numerous pores or fenestrations, which allow for the efficient exchange of substances between the blood and hepatocytes. These fenestrations are larger than those found in typical capillaries.

Blood Flow: Blood flows slowly through liver sinusoids, allowing for extended contact between the blood and hepatocytes. This is important for the liver's metabolic and detoxification functions.

Nutrient Exchange: Liver sinusoids play a central role in the exchange of nutrients, oxygen, and waste products between the bloodstream and hepatocytes. Nutrients absorbed from the digestive tract, carried by the hepatic portal vein, pass through sinusoids and are processed by hepatocytes.

Detoxification: Liver sinusoids facilitate the removal of toxins, drugs, and metabolic waste products from the bloodstream. Hepatocytes within the lobules can metabolize and neutralize harmful substances before they continue in the circulation.

Phagocytosis: Specialized macrophages called Kupffer cells are located within the sinusoids. They play a role in phagocytosing (engulfing and digesting) pathogens, bacteria, and foreign particles that enter the liver through the bloodstream.

Bile Production: Bile canaliculi, small ducts formed by hepatocytes, transport bile produced by the liver to the bile ducts. These canaliculi connect to the bile ducts within the liver lobules, allowing for the secretion of bile into bile ducts and eventual storage in the gallbladder.

In summary, liver sinusoids are critical to the liver's function as they enable the efficient exchange of nutrients, oxygen, and waste products between the blood and hepatocytes. Their unique structure and slow blood flow contribute to the liver's metabolic, detoxification, and secretory activities, making the liver a central organ for maintaining metabolic and overall physiological balance in the body.

Hepatic veins

Hepatic veins are a system of veins responsible for draining deoxygenated blood from the liver and returning it to the systemic circulation. These veins play a vital role in completing the liver's circulatory function. Here are some key points about hepatic veins:

Origin: Hepatic veins originate within the liver, specifically within the liver lobules. They collect blood that has been processed and filtered by hepatocytes (liver cells) within the liver sinusoids.

Convergence: Several smaller hepatic veins within the liver combine and merge into larger hepatic veins as they progress toward the liver's posterior surface.

Inferior Vena Cava (IVC): The hepatic veins ultimately converge into the inferior vena cava (IVC), a large vein that carries deoxygenated blood from the lower half of the body back to the heart. The point where the hepatic veins join the IVC is located just below the diaphragm on the right side of the body.

Blood Flow: Hepatic veins carry deoxygenated blood, as well as metabolic waste products and nutrients processed by the liver, away from the liver tissue. This blood then enters the right atrium of the heart, where it is subsequently pumped into the lungs for oxygenation.

Function: The hepatic veins, along with the hepatic portal vein and hepatic artery, complete the liver's circulatory system. They help regulate the distribution of nutrients and oxygen to the liver while ensuring that processed blood is returned to the general circulation for use by other tissues and organs.

Hepatic veins are responsible for draining deoxygenated blood from the liver and returning it to the systemic circulation. This process is essential for maintaining overall blood flow and metabolic balance within the body.

Chapter 7: Biliary System

Structure of bile ducts

The bile ducts are a network of tubes and ducts that transport bile from the liver and gallbladder to the small intestine, where it aids in digestion. These ducts have a specific structure designed for the efficient transport of bile. Here are the main components and characteristics of the structure of bile ducts:

Hepatic Ducts: Bile is initially produced by the liver and flows into small ducts called hepatic ducts within the liver. There are typically two hepatic ducts: the right hepatic duct and the left hepatic duct, which originate from the right and left lobes of the liver, respectively.

Intrahepatic Bile Ducts: These are the bile ducts found within the liver. They collect bile produced by hepatocytes (liver cells) and transport it toward the outside of the liver. Intrahepatic bile ducts progressively merge to form larger ducts.

Common Hepatic Duct: The right and left hepatic ducts merge to form a single common hepatic duct. This common hepatic duct carries bile out of the liver and toward the gallbladder or the small intestine.

Gallbladder (Optional): If the gallbladder is present, the common hepatic duct may join with the cystic duct, which comes from the gallbladder. The point of connection is known as the common bile duct.

Common Bile Duct: The common bile duct is the main conduit for bile transport. It carries bile from both the liver and the gallbladder, if applicable, towards the small intestine. It can also release bile into the duodenum (the first part of the small intestine) when needed for digestion.

Cystic Duct: The cystic duct connects the gallbladder to the common bile duct. When the gallbladder contracts, bile flows from the gallbladder into the cystic duct and then into the common bile duct.

Pancreatic Duct (Optional): In some individuals, the common bile duct may merge with the pancreatic duct just before entering the duodenum. This junction is called the hepatopancreatic ampulla, or the ampulla of Vater. The pancreatic duct carries digestive enzymes from the pancreas.

Sphincters: At the junction of the common bile duct and the pancreatic duct, there are sphincters that control the release of bile and pancreatic enzymes into the duodenum. The sphincter of Oddi controls the flow of both bile and pancreatic enzymes.

Duodenal Papilla: The common bile duct opens into the duodenum (the first part of the small intestine) at a small, nipple-like structure called the duodenal papilla. Here, bile is released into the digestive tract to aid in the digestion and absorption of fats.

Mucosa and Epithelial Lining: The inner lining of the bile ducts is composed of mucosa with specialized epithelial cells. These cells help transport bile and regulate its composition.

The structure of bile ducts allows for the regulated transport of bile from the liver and, if necessary, from the gallbladder to the small intestine. Bile plays a critical role in emulsifying fats and aiding in their digestion and absorption in the digestive tract.

Gallbladder and its function

- Is located at the junction of the right ninth costal cartilage and lateral border of the rectus abdominis, which is the site of maximum tenderness in acute inflammation of the gallbladder.
- Is a pear-shaped sac lying on the inferior surface of the liver in a fossa between the right and quadrate lobes with a capacity of approximately 30 to 50 mL and is in contact with the duodenum and transverse colon.
- Consists of the fundus, body, and neck: the fundus is the rounded blind end located at the tip of the right ninth costal cartilage in the midclavicular line and contacts the transverse colon; the body is the major part and rests on the upper part of the duodenum and the transverse

colon; the neck is the narrow part and gives rise to the cystic duct with spiral valves (Heister's valves).

- Receives bile, concentrates it (by absorbing water and salts), stores it, and releases it during digestion.
- Contracts to expel bile as a result of stimulation by the hormone cholecystokinin, which is produced by the duodenal mucosa or by parasympathetic stimulation when food arrives in the duodenum.
- Receives blood from the cystic artery, which arises from the right hepatic artery within the cystohepatic triangle (of Calot), which is formed by the visceral surface of the liver superiorly, the cystic duct inferiorly, and the common hepatic duct medially.
- May have an abnormal conical pouch (Hartmann's pouch) in its neck and the pouch is also called the ampulla of the gallbladder.

Bile production and transport

Bile production and transport are essential processes in the digestive system, particularly in the breakdown and absorption of dietary fats. Here's an overview of how bile is produced and transported in the body:

Bile Production:

Hepatocytes (Liver Cells): The production of bile begins in the liver, where specialized cells called hepatocytes synthesize bile from cholesterol, bile salts, bilirubin (a breakdown product of red blood cells), and other components.

Bile Secretion: Hepatocytes continuously secrete bile into small bile ducts within the liver known as intrahepatic bile ducts. The bile produced by hepatocytes contains bile salts and other substances necessary for fat digestion.

Bile Modification: As bile moves through the intrahepatic bile ducts, it undergoes modification, including the addition of bicarbonate ions to neutralize its acidity.

Storage in the Gallbladder: Bile flows from the intrahepatic bile ducts into the common hepatic duct, and from there, it enters the common bile duct. A portion of this bile is diverted into the gallbladder for storage and concentration.

Bile Transport:

Gallbladder Storage: In the gallbladder, bile is stored and concentrated. When you consume a meal that contains fats, the gallbladder contracts in response to hormonal signals, releasing the concentrated bile.

Common Bile Duct: The bile released from the gallbladder flows into the common bile duct, which combines with the common hepatic duct from the liver.

Duodenal Papilla: The common bile duct opens into the duodenum (the first part of the small intestine) at a small, nipple-like structure called the duodenal papilla. Here, bile is released into the digestive tract to aid in the digestion and absorption of fats.

Sphincter of Oddi: The sphincter of Oddi, a muscular valve located at the junction of the common bile duct and the duodenum, regulates the release of bile into the small intestine. It ensures that bile is delivered when needed for fat digestion.

Bile is produced in the liver by hepatocytes, modified as it moves through bile ducts within the liver, stored and concentrated in the gallbladder, and released into the small intestine when fats are present in the digestive tract. Bile plays a crucial role in emulsifying fats, making them accessible for digestion by enzymes, and aiding in the absorption of fat-soluble nutrients.

Chapter 8: Liver Functions

Metabolism of Nutrients

The liver is a central hub for the metabolism of nutrients in the body, and it plays a pivotal role in regulating various metabolic processes. Here's a concise overview of how the liver metabolizes key nutrients:

Carbohydrate Metabolism:

Glycogen Storage: The liver stores excess glucose as glycogen when blood sugar levels are high, primarily after a meal. When blood sugar levels drop, the liver can break down glycogen into glucose and release it into the bloodstream to maintain stable blood sugar levels.

Gluconeogenesis: The liver can also synthesize glucose from non-carbohydrate sources, such as amino acids and glycerol, through a process called gluconeogenesis. This is important for maintaining blood glucose levels during fasting.

Lipid Metabolism:

Lipogenesis: The liver can synthesize lipids (fats) from excess glucose and other precursors. These lipids can be stored in adipose tissue or transported to other tissues for energy.

Lipolysis: The liver can break down stored fats and release fatty acids into the bloodstream for energy production.

Protein Metabolism:

Protein Synthesis: The liver synthesizes many essential proteins, including blood clotting factors, albumin, and enzymes involved in various metabolic processes.

Amino Acid Metabolism: The liver plays a key role in the metabolism of amino acids. It can convert one amino acid into another and remove excess nitrogen from amino acids through the process of deamination.

Detoxification:

The liver detoxifies harmful substances, such as drugs, alcohol, and metabolic waste products, by converting them into less toxic or water-soluble compounds that can be excreted from the body.

Storage of Nutrients:

The liver stores essential nutrients like vitamins (e.g., vitamin A, D, B12) and minerals (e.g., iron) for later use.

Regulation of Nutrient Levels:

The liver regulates the levels of nutrients in the bloodstream, ensuring a steady supply of essential substances to various tissues and organs.

Bile Production: The liver produces bile, which is essential for the digestion and absorption of dietary fats and fat-soluble vitamins in the small intestine.

The liver plays a central role in metabolizing carbohydrates, lipids, and proteins, regulating nutrient levels, and detoxifying the body. Its multifaceted functions are crucial for maintaining metabolic balance and overall health.

Detoxification and Toxin Removal

The liver is a vital organ responsible for detoxifying the body and removing harmful substances. Here's a concise explanation of how the liver performs detoxification and toxin removal:

Metabolic Detoxification:

The liver metabolizes and neutralizes various toxins, drugs, and metabolic waste products that enter the bloodstream. This process involves enzymes that convert these substances into less toxic or water-soluble forms.

Phase I and Phase II Reactions:

Detoxification occurs in two phases: Phase I and Phase II.

- Phase I reactions involve the modification of toxins, often by adding functional groups to make them more water-soluble. This can make them easier to eliminate.

- Phase II reactions involve the conjugation of toxins with molecules like glutathione, sulfate, or glycine. Conjugation makes toxins more water-soluble and facilitates their removal from the body.

Bile Production and Excretion:

The liver produces bile, which contains conjugated toxins and waste products. Bile is transported to the small intestine and released into the digestive tract. From there, these toxins can be eliminated from the body through feces.

Kupffer Cells:

Kupffer cells are specialized macrophages located in the liver sinusoids. They play a role in the immune system and assist in removing bacteria, pathogens, and damaged blood cells from the bloodstream, contributing to detoxification.

Alcohol Metabolism:

The liver metabolizes alcohol (ethanol) into acetaldehyde and then further into acetic acid, which is less toxic. This process helps the body eliminate alcohol.

Drug Metabolism:

The liver processes and metabolizes drugs, rendering them less toxic and more suitable for elimination from the body. This is an essential function in drug metabolism and pharmaceutical safety.

Ammonia Conversion:

The liver converts toxic ammonia, a byproduct of protein metabolism, into urea, which is excreted in urine.

Storage of Toxins:

The liver can temporarily store certain toxins to prevent them from immediately circulating in the bloodstream. This storage helps to limit the potential harm to other organs.

Storage of Vitamins and Minerals

The liver plays a significant role in the storage of vitamins and minerals, helping to regulate their availability to the body as needed. Here's how the liver is involved in the storage of these essential nutrients:

Vitamins:

   Vitamin A: The liver stores vitamin A in the form of retinyl esters. When the body requires vitamin A for functions such as vision, immune health, and skin health, the liver releases it into the bloodstream.

   Vitamin D: The liver converts vitamin D obtained from sunlight or dietary sources into its active form, calcitriol. The liver can store some vitamin D, releasing it when necessary to support calcium absorption and bone health.

Vitamin B12: The liver stores significant amounts of vitamin B12. It releases this vitamin into the bloodstream when needed for functions such as red blood cell production, neurological health, and DNA synthesis.

Vitamin K: The liver stores vitamin K, which is essential for blood clotting and bone health. It releases vitamin K into the bloodstream to support these functions.

Minerals:

Iron: The liver stores excess iron as ferritin. When the body requires iron for the production of red blood cells or other functions, the liver releases it into the bloodstream.

Copper: The liver stores copper and regulates its release into the bloodstream. Copper is essential for various metabolic processes, including the formation of connective tissue and the production of energy.

Zinc: The liver plays a role in the storage and release of zinc, which is important for immune function, wound healing, and DNA synthesis.

Selenium: The liver stores selenium and releases it when needed for antioxidant defense and thyroid hormone metabolism.

Function of Storage:

- The liver's ability to store these vitamins and minerals ensures a continuous and stable supply of these essential nutrients to the body, even when dietary intake may be insufficient.
- When the body needs these nutrients, the liver can release them into the bloodstream as required, helping to maintain overall nutritional balance.
- This storage function is especially valuable during periods of dietary deficiency or increased demand for these nutrients, such as during illness or pregnancy.

The liver acts as a storage reservoir for these vitamins and minerals, ensuring that the body has a consistent supply even when dietary intake fluctuates. This storage and release mechanism helps maintain the overall balance and homeostasis of essential nutrients in the body, supporting various physiological processes and overall health.

Synthesis of Proteins, Including Clotting Factors

The liver is a major site for the synthesis of various proteins, including clotting factors. Here's an overview of the synthesis of proteins, particularly clotting factors, in the liver:

Clotting Factors Synthesis:

The liver synthesizes several clotting factors, including fibrinogen, prothrombin, and factors I (fibrinogen), II (prothrombin), V, VII, IX, X, XI, and XII.

These clotting factors are essential for the blood clotting cascade, which is a series of enzymatic reactions that prevent excessive bleeding after injury.

Albumin:

The liver produces a significant amount of albumin, a protein that helps maintain osmotic pressure in the blood, regulates fluid balance, and transports various substances, including hormones, drugs, and fatty acids.

Transferrin:

Transferrin, synthesized in the liver, plays a crucial role in transporting iron in the bloodstream. It binds to iron and delivers it to cells and tissues, including bone marrow for red blood cell production.

Alpha and Beta Globulins:

The liver produces various alpha and beta globulins, including alpha-1 antitrypsin and beta-2 microglobulin, which are involved in immune function and maintaining protein balance in the blood.

Other Proteins:

The liver synthesizes numerous other proteins, such as lipoproteins (involved in lipid transport), acute-phase proteins (responding to inflammation), and complement proteins (part of the immune system).

Synthesis Process:

- Hepatocytes (liver cells) are primarily responsible for protein synthesis in the liver. These cells contain abundant ribosomes and endoplasmic reticulum, which are essential for protein production.
- The process of protein synthesis involves transcription and translation of genetic information stored in DNA.
- Once synthesized, proteins are released into the bloodstream and transported to various target tissues and organs where they perform their specific functions.

Overall, the liver's ability to synthesize proteins, including clotting factors, is vital for maintaining the body's overall health and ensuring proper blood clotting, immune function, and transport of essential substances. Liver diseases or conditions that affect liver function can disrupt protein synthesis and lead to various health issues.

Chapter 9: Innervation

Nerves and ganglia

The liver is primarily composed of hepatocytes (liver cells) and other specialized cells, and it doesn't have a significant presence of nerves or ganglia within its tissue. However, it is indirectly connected to the nervous system through the following mechanisms:

Autonomic Nervous System (ANS): The liver receives sympathetic and parasympathetic nerve fibers from the autonomic nervous system, which regulates various physiological processes, including blood flow to the liver, bile secretion, and metabolic activity. These nerves don't form ganglia within the liver but control liver function through neural signaling.

Plexuses and Ganglia Nearby: The liver is located in the upper right abdomen, adjacent to the celiac plexus and the coeliac ganglia. These autonomic nerve structures serve nearby organs like the stomach, pancreas, and small intestine. While they are not within the liver tissue itself, they can indirectly influence liver function.

Hepatic Innervation: The hepatic artery and portal vein, which supply the liver with blood, also carry sympathetic and parasympathetic nerves. These nerves help regulate blood flow, nutrient supply, and metabolic activity in the liver.

Pain Sensation: While the liver itself doesn't have sensory nerves for pain perception, the liver capsule, a thin layer surrounding the liver, is innervated by sensory nerves. In cases of liver inflammation or stretching of the liver capsule, pain signals can be transmitted to the central nervous system, leading to abdominal discomfort or pain.

The liver does not contain a complex network of nerves or ganglia within its tissue. Instead, it is regulated by the autonomic nervous system, which indirectly influences liver function through neural signaling. Pain and discomfort related to liver conditions may be sensed through sensory nerves in the liver capsule.

Autonomic control of liver functions

The autonomic nervous system (ANS) plays a significant role in regulating various liver functions. The liver is innervated by both sympathetic and parasympathetic nerves, and the balance between these two divisions of the ANS helps maintain homeostasis and control liver activities. Here's how the ANS influences liver functions:

Sympathetic Nervous System:

The sympathetic nerves that innervate the liver originate from the celiac ganglia and travel along the hepatic artery.

Sympathetic stimulation typically leads to:

- Constriction of blood vessels (vasoconstriction) in the liver, which can reduce blood flow to the liver.
- Inhibition of bile secretion.
- **Glycogenolysis:** The breakdown of glycogen into glucose, leading to an increase in blood sugar levels. This can provide energy during the "fight or flight" response.

- Inhibition of non-essential metabolic processes in the liver to prioritize energy conservation for other bodily functions.

Parasympathetic Nervous System:

The parasympathetic nerves that innervate the liver arise from the vagus nerve (cranial nerve X) and synapse in the liver.

Parasympathetic stimulation typically leads to:

- Vasodilation of blood vessels in the liver, increasing blood flow to support metabolic activities.
- Stimulation of bile secretion, facilitating digestion and the absorption of fats.
- **Promotion of glycogenesis:** The conversion of glucose into glycogen for storage, which helps lower blood sugar levels.
- Facilitation of various metabolic and digestive processes in the liver.

Balance and Regulation:

- The liver's functions are finely tuned through the balance of sympathetic and parasympathetic input.
- The liver responds to neural signals to adapt to changing metabolic demands. For example, after a meal, parasympathetic activity may dominate to support digestion and nutrient processing, while sympathetic activity may increase during periods of stress or physical activity.

The autonomic nervous system regulates liver functions by controlling blood flow, bile secretion, and metabolic processes such as glucose storage and release. This intricate neural regulation allows the liver to adapt to the body's changing needs and maintain overall metabolic homeostasis.

Role in digestion and metabolism

The liver plays a crucial role in digestion and metabolism:

Digestion: The liver produces bile, which emulsifies fats, making them easier to digest in the small intestine. Bile also aids in the absorption of fat-soluble vitamins.

Metabolism: The liver metabolizes carbohydrates, fats, and proteins. It stores and releases glucose to maintain blood sugar levels, converts excess nutrients into storage forms, and detoxifies harmful substances from the body.

In short, the liver's functions support the digestion of nutrients and regulate metabolic processes to ensure the body's energy needs are met and toxins are removed.

Chapter 10: Liver Development

Embryological development of the liver

The embryological development of the liver is a complex process that takes place during early fetal development. Here's a simplified overview of the key stages and events in the embryological development of the liver:

Endoderm Formation:

The liver, like many other digestive organs, originates from the endoderm, one of the primary germ layers in the developing embryo.

Formation of the Liver Bud:

Around the third week of embryonic development, a structure called the hepatic diverticulum or liver bud begins to form from the endoderm. This bud emerges from the developing gut tube.

Growth and Differentiation:

The liver bud undergoes rapid growth and differentiation, giving rise to the hepatoblasts. Hepatoblasts are precursor cells that will eventually develop into hepatocytes (mature liver cells) and cholangiocytes (cells lining the bile ducts).

Vascularization:

As the liver continues to grow, it becomes highly vascularized. Blood vessels, including the hepatic artery and portal vein, develop to supply the growing organ.

Bile Duct Formation:

Simultaneously, the bile ducts develop from the hepatoblasts, forming a network of ducts that will transport bile produced by the liver.

Formation of Liver Lobes:

The liver undergoes further growth and structural organization, leading to the formation of the two primary liver lobes: the right lobe and the left lobe.

These lobes are initially separated by the developing gallbladder.

Functional Maturation:

As the liver matures, it becomes increasingly involved in metabolic functions, including the production of enzymes, proteins, and bile. These functions are essential for supporting the developing embryo's metabolic needs.

Functional Integration:

The liver becomes integrated with other developing digestive organs, including the pancreas, gallbladder, and intestines. These organs work together to support digestion, nutrient absorption, and waste elimination.

The embryological development of the liver is a highly orchestrated process that ensures the formation of a functional organ with a complex structure and the ability to perform vital metabolic and digestive functions after birth. Any disruptions or abnormalities during this developmental process can lead to congenital liver disorders.

Changes throughout life

The liver undergoes various changes throughout a person's life, adapting to different stages of growth, development, and aging. Here's an overview of the key liver changes at different life stages:

Fetal and Neonatal Period:

- In the fetal stage, the liver is a crucial site for the production of blood cells (hematopoiesis).
- After birth, the liver continues to play a vital role in metabolizing nutrients from breast milk or formula.

Infancy and Childhood:

- The liver continues to grow and develop, adapting to the changing nutritional needs of the growing child.
- It matures in terms of enzymatic functions, allowing for the digestion and absorption of solid foods as the child transitions from a liquid diet.

Adolescence and Young Adulthood:

- The liver continues to support the rapid growth and development seen during these years.
- Metabolic functions, including carbohydrate and fat metabolism, are fully established, and the liver is involved in hormone regulation.

Adulthood:

- The liver maintains its metabolic functions, including the processing of nutrients, detoxification of drugs and toxins, and the synthesis of proteins.
- The liver is capable of regenerating damaged tissue to a certain extent, which helps it recover from injuries and maintain its functionality.

Aging:

- With age, there can be a gradual decline in liver size and blood flow.
- The liver's regenerative capacity may decrease, making it more vulnerable to injury or disease.

- Accumulation of fat in the liver (fatty liver) may become more common in older adults, potentially leading to liver-related health issues.
- Liver diseases, such as hepatitis and cirrhosis, may become more prevalent in older age, affecting liver function.

Overall Adaptation:

- Throughout life, the liver adapts to various dietary and metabolic challenges.
- It continues to produce bile, support digestion, and maintain metabolic balance.
- The liver's ability to metabolize drugs may change, affecting medication dosages required as a person ages.

Gender-Specific Changes:

- In females, hormonal changes during puberty, pregnancy, and menopause can influence liver function.

- In males, factors such as alcohol consumption and exposure to toxins may impact the liver differently at various life stages.

It's important to note that lifestyle choices, such as diet, alcohol consumption, and exposure to toxins, can significantly impact liver health at any age. Regular medical check-ups and a healthy lifestyle can help ensure that the liver functions optimally throughout life. Additionally, liver health can be influenced by genetics and underlying medical conditions.

Chapter 11: Common Liver Conditions

Hepatitis

Hepatitis refers to inflammation of the liver, which can be caused by various factors, including viral infections. There are several types of viral hepatitis, each caused by different hepatitis viruses. The most common types of viral hepatitis include:

Hepatitis A (HAV):

Transmission: Primarily through contaminated food or water, and occasionally through close person-to-person contact.

Acute Infection: Typically results in acute hepatitis with symptoms such as fever, jaundice, fatigue, and abdominal pain.

Vaccine: Available and highly effective in preventing hepatitis A.

Hepatitis B (HBV):

Transmission: Through contact with infected blood, unprotected sex, sharing needles, or from an infected mother to her newborn during childbirth.

Acute and Chronic Infection: Can cause acute hepatitis, but many cases progress to chronic infection, which can lead to cirrhosis and liver cancer.

Vaccine: Available and recommended for routine immunization.

Hepatitis C (HCV):

Transmission: Primarily through contact with infected blood, often through sharing needles or receiving contaminated medical procedures.

Chronic Infection: Most cases of hepatitis C become chronic, potentially leading to liver cirrhosis and cancer.

No Vaccine: There is currently no vaccine for hepatitis C, but antiviral treatments are available.

Hepatitis D (HDV):

Transmission: Only occurs in individuals who are already infected with hepatitis B. HDV is a defective virus that requires the presence of HBV to replicate.

Chronic Infection: Can lead to chronic hepatitis, often more severe than hepatitis B alone.

Prevention: Hepatitis B vaccination can also prevent hepatitis D in those not previously infected with HBV.

Hepatitis E (HEV):

Transmission: Similar to hepatitis A, primarily through contaminated food and water.

Acute Infection: Most cases result in acute hepatitis with symptoms, but it can be severe, especially in pregnant women.

No Vaccine: Limited availability of vaccines, primarily in certain regions.

Autoimmune Hepatitis:

Not caused by a viral infection but rather an autoimmune response where the body's immune system attacks the liver.

Chronic Disease: Can lead to chronic hepatitis and cirrhosis if not properly managed.

Alcoholic Hepatitis:

Caused by excessive alcohol consumption over an extended period.

Can range from mild inflammation to severe liver damage (alcoholic liver disease).

Non-Alcoholic Fatty Liver Disease (NAFLD):

Associated with obesity, diabetes, and metabolic syndrome.

Can progress from simple fat accumulation in the liver (steatosis) to non-alcoholic steatohepatitis (NASH) and liver fibrosis.

It's important to note that hepatitis viruses differ in terms of transmission, acute and chronic outcomes, and available prevention measures. Vaccines are available for hepatitis A and B and are important tools for preventing these infections. Treatment options vary depending on the type of hepatitis and the stage of the disease. Early diagnosis and management are essential to prevent liver damage and complications.

Cirrhosis

Cirrhosis is a late stage of scarring (fibrosis) of the liver caused by many forms of liver diseases and conditions, such as hepatitis and chronic alcoholism. The liver carries out several necessary functions, including detoxifying harmful substances in your body, cleaning your blood, and making vital nutrients. Cirrhosis can lead to a number of complications, including liver cancer.

Cirrhosis occurs in response to damage to your liver. Each time your liver is injured, it tries to repair itself. In the process, scar tissue forms. As the cirrhosis progresses, more and more scar tissue forms, making it difficult for the liver to function.

Complications of cirrhosis can include:

Fluid buildup in the abdomen (ascites): The liver makes albumin, a protein that helps keep the blood vessels from leaking fluid. Cirrhosis decreases your liver's ability to make albumin. Fluid may build up in your abdomen and legs (edema).

Swelling in the legs and ankles (edema): Fluid buildup in the legs and ankles can occur as the liver loses its ability to function properly.

Enlargement of the spleen (splenomegaly): Portal hypertension can cause the spleen to enlarge and hold on to more platelets than it normally would.

Infections: People with cirrhosis are at risk of a type of serious bacterial infection called spontaneous bacterial peritonitis.

Bleeding: Cirrhosis can lead to a bleeding disorder. This can cause you to bruise or bleed easily, often from the esophagus, stomach, or intestines.

Confusion, drowsiness and slurred speech (hepatic encephalopathy): A liver damaged by cirrhosis isn't able to clear toxins from the blood as well as a healthy liver can. These toxins can then build up in the brain and cause mental confusion and difficulty concentrating.

Kidney and lung problems: Cirrhosis can lead to kidney and lung failure.

Liver cancer: A damaged liver is more likely to develop cancer.

The liver damage done by cirrhosis generally can't be undone, but if liver cirrhosis is diagnosed early and the cause is treated, further damage and complications can be limited and reduced.

Liver cancer

Liver cancer is a serious medical condition that occurs when malignant cells develop in the liver. It can be primary (originating in the liver) or secondary (resulting from the spread of cancer from other parts of the body). Common risk factors include chronic hepatitis B or C infection, cirrhosis, alcohol abuse, and certain genetic conditions. Treatment options may include surgery, radiation therapy, chemotherapy, targeted therapy, or liver transplantation, depending on the stage and type of liver cancer. Early detection and intervention are crucial for better outcomes. If you have concerns about liver cancer, it's important to consult with a healthcare professional.

Stages of liver cancer

Liver cancer, also known as hepatocellular carcinoma (HCC), is typically staged using the Barcelona Clinic Liver Cancer (BCLC) staging system or the TNM (Tumor, Node, Metastasis) system. Here's an overview of the BCLC stages:

1. BCLC Stage 0:

   - Very early-stage HCC.

   - Single tumor smaller than 2 cm in size.

   - No evidence of cirrhosis or portal hypertension.

   - Good liver function.

2. BCLC Stage A:

   - Early-stage HCC.

   - A single tumor or a few small tumors.

   - May or may not have cirrhosis, but liver function is preserved.

3. BCLC Stage B:

 - Intermediate-stage HCC.

 - Multiple tumors or a larger tumor.

 - May have spread to nearby blood vessels.

 - Liver function might be slightly impaired.

4. BCLC Stage C:

 - Advanced-stage HCC.

 - The cancer has spread extensively within the liver or to nearby lymph nodes.

 - Liver function is often impaired.

5. BCLC Stage D:

   - End-stage HCC.

   - The cancer has spread to distant organs or to other parts of the body.

   - Liver function is severely compromised.

It's important to note that the choice of treatment and prognosis can vary depending on the stage of liver cancer. Early detection and treatment are crucial for better outcomes, so regular screening and early intervention are recommended for individuals at risk. Please consult with a healthcare professional for personalized information and treatment options.

Hepatic tumors

Liver tumors can be broadly categorized into two main types: benign and malignant.

Benign Liver Tumors: These are non-cancerous growths that develop in the liver. Some common types include:

Hemangiomas: These are made up of blood vessels and are usually harmless.

Hepatic adenomas: These are rare and may require removal if they cause symptoms or are at risk of rupture.

Focal nodular hyperplasia (FNH): FNH is usually benign and typically doesn't require treatment unless it causes symptoms.

Malignant Liver Tumors: These are cancerous growths that can be primary (originating in the liver) or secondary (metastatic tumors that have spread from other parts of the body). The most common primary liver cancer is hepatocellular carcinoma

(HCC). Other primary liver cancers include cholangiocarcinoma and angiosarcoma. Secondary liver tumors, also known as metastatic liver cancer, are more common than primary liver cancers and can originate from various organs, such as the colon, lung, or breast.

Symptoms of liver tumors may include abdominal pain, unexplained weight loss, jaundice (yellowing of the skin and eyes), and abdominal swelling. Diagnosis often involves imaging tests like CT scans or MRI, and a biopsy may be needed to confirm if a tumor is cancerous.

The treatment of liver tumors depends on their type, size, location, and stage. Options may include surgery, liver transplantation, ablation therapy, chemotherapy, radiation therapy, and targeted therapy. The choice of treatment is made on a case-by-case basis after careful evaluation by a medical team.

Liver abscess

A liver abscess is a localized collection of pus within the liver. It can be caused by various factors, including:

Bacterial Infections: The most common cause of liver abscesses is a bacterial infection, often stemming from an infection elsewhere in the body that spreads to the liver through the bloodstream. The bacteria most frequently associated with liver abscesses are Escherichia coli and Klebsiella.

Amoebic Infections: In some regions, particularly in developing countries, liver abscesses can be caused by a parasite called Entamoeba histolytica, leading to amoebic liver abscess.

Trauma: Liver trauma, such as a penetrating injury, can introduce bacteria into the liver and lead to abscess formation.

Biliary Tract Infections: Infections in the biliary system, such as cholecystitis or cholangitis, can sometimes lead to liver abscesses.

Symptoms of a liver abscess may include fever, abdominal pain in the upper right quadrant, jaundice (yellowing of the skin and eyes), nausea, vomiting, and general malaise.

Treatment typically involves antibiotics to combat the underlying infection and may also include draining the abscess. The method of drainage (percutaneous, surgical, or endoscopic) depends on the size and location of the abscess. Liver abscesses can be a serious medical condition, and prompt diagnosis and treatment are essential to prevent complications. If you suspect you have a liver abscess or are experiencing symptoms, it's important to seek medical attention.

Fatty liver disease

Fatty liver disease, also known as hepatic steatosis, is a condition characterized by the accumulation of excess fat in the liver cells. There are two main types of fatty liver disease:

Non-Alcoholic Fatty Liver Disease (NAFLD): This is the most common form and is not related to alcohol consumption. NAFLD can range from simple fatty liver (steatosis) to a more severe condition known as non-alcoholic steatohepatitis (NASH), which involves inflammation and liver cell damage. NASH can progress to cirrhosis and liver failure over time.

Alcoholic Fatty Liver Disease: This condition is caused by excessive alcohol consumption and is characterized by the accumulation of fat in the liver due to the toxic effects of alcohol. It can progress to more severe liver conditions like alcoholic hepatitis and cirrhosis.

Risk factors for fatty liver disease include obesity, type 2 diabetes, insulin resistance, high blood pressure, high cholesterol levels, rapid weight loss, and certain medications. The exact cause of NAFLD is not fully understood but is thought to be related to a combination of genetic, metabolic, and lifestyle factors.

Symptoms of fatty liver disease are often absent or mild in the early stages. However, as the disease progresses, individuals may experience symptoms such as fatigue, abdominal discomfort, and hepatomegaly (enlarged liver). The condition is often discovered incidentally through blood tests or imaging studies.

Management of fatty liver disease typically involves lifestyle changes, including:

- Weight loss through a healthy diet and exercise, as obesity is a significant risk factor.
- Avoiding excessive alcohol consumption.
- Managing underlying conditions like diabetes and high cholesterol.
- Regular monitoring and follow-up with a healthcare provider.

In severe cases, especially with NASH or advanced alcoholic liver disease, medical treatment and specialized care may be necessary. Early diagnosis and intervention are essential in preventing the progression of fatty liver disease to more severe liver conditions. If you suspect you may have fatty liver disease or are at risk, it's important to consult a healthcare professional for evaluation and guidance.

Chapter 12: Diagnostic Techniques

Imaging methods

Imaging studies of the liver are essential for diagnosing and evaluating various liver conditions, including liver diseases, tumors, and abnormalities. Here are some common imaging techniques used to examine the liver:

Ultrasound (US): Ultrasound is a widely used and non-invasive imaging method. It uses high-frequency sound waves to create real-time images of the liver and surrounding structures. It is helpful in detecting liver abnormalities, such as fatty liver, cysts, and tumors.

Computed Tomography (CT) Scan: CT scans use X-rays and computer technology to produce detailed cross-sectional images of the liver. It can provide information about liver size, shape, and the presence of tumors, abscesses, or other abnormalities. Contrast agents may be used to enhance the images.

Magnetic Resonance Imaging (MRI): MRI utilizes powerful magnets and radio waves to create detailed images of the liver. It is particularly useful for detecting liver tumors, characterizing lesions, and assessing liver function. Contrast agents can be used in MRI as well.

CT or MRI Angiography: These specialized imaging techniques focus on the blood vessels in and around the liver. They are used to assess the blood supply to liver tumors, identify vascular abnormalities, and plan interventions like embolization or surgery.

Fibroscan (Transient Elastography): This is a specialized ultrasound-based technique used to assess liver fibrosis (scarring) and stiffness. It's often used to evaluate liver damage in individuals with chronic liver diseases like hepatitis and cirrhosis.

Nuclear Medicine Scans: Certain nuclear medicine scans, such as a liver/spleen scan or a hepatobiliary iminodiacetic acid (HIDA) scan, can provide functional information about liver and bile duct function.

Positron Emission Tomography (PET) Scan: PET scans are used to detect areas of increased metabolic activity in the liver, which can be indicative of liver tumors or metastasis from other parts of the body.

The choice of imaging study depends on the specific clinical situation and the information needed by the healthcare provider to make a diagnosis or plan treatment. Imaging studies of the liver play a crucial role in early detection, diagnosis, and monitoring of liver diseases, helping healthcare professionals provide appropriate care to patients.

Blood tests

Blood tests to assess liver function and health are an essential part of diagnosing and monitoring various liver conditions. Here are some common blood tests used to evaluate the liver:

Liver Function Tests (LFTs): These tests include several markers that provide information about the overall health and function of the liver. Key LFTs include:

- **Alanine Aminotransferase (ALT):** Elevated ALT levels may indicate liver damage or inflammation, often associated with conditions like hepatitis.
- **Aspartate Aminotransferase (AST):** Like ALT, elevated AST levels can indicate liver injury, although it is found in other organs as well.
- **Alkaline Phosphatase (ALP):** Elevated ALP can be a sign of liver or bile duct problems.
- **Total Bilirubin:** Bilirubin is a waste product that can accumulate in the blood when the liver isn't processing it properly. Elevated levels can cause jaundice.
- **Albumin:** Albumin is a protein produced by the liver. Low levels may suggest liver disease or malnutrition.

Liver Enzymes: Apart from ALT and AST, there are other liver enzymes, like gamma-glutamyl transferase (GGT), that can be elevated in liver conditions, particularly when related to alcohol abuse or biliary problems.

Prothrombin Time (PT) and International Normalized Ratio (INR): These tests measure the blood's ability to clot. Abnormal results can indicate liver damage or impaired liver function, as the liver plays a crucial role in blood clotting.

Serum Protein Electrophoresis: This test assesses the types and levels of proteins in the blood, including specific proteins produced by the liver. Changes in protein patterns can indicate liver disease.

Viral Hepatitis Markers: Blood tests can detect antibodies or viral genetic material associated with hepatitis viruses (e.g., hepatitis A, B, C) to diagnose and monitor these infections.

Liver Panel: A comprehensive panel of liver tests may be ordered, combining several of the above markers to provide a broader view of liver health.

Fibrosis Markers: In some cases, specialized tests like FibroTest or FibroScan may be used to assess the degree of liver fibrosis (scarring) caused by conditions like hepatitis or cirrhosis.

The interpretation of these blood test results depends on the specific markers, the patient's medical history, and other clinical information. Abnormal results may indicate various liver disorders, including hepatitis, cirrhosis, fatty liver disease, or tumors. Early detection through blood tests can be crucial for effective management and treatment of liver conditions.

Biopsy

A liver biopsy is a medical procedure in which a small sample of liver tissue is collected for examination under a microscope. It is typically performed when there is a need to diagnose or evaluate various liver conditions, including liver diseases, tumors, fibrosis, or inflammation. There are different methods for obtaining a liver biopsy:

Percutaneous Liver Biopsy: This is the most common method. It involves inserting a thin, hollow needle through the skin and into the liver to collect a small tissue sample. It is usually guided by ultrasound or other imaging techniques to ensure accurate placement of the needle.

Transjugular Liver Biopsy: In this approach, a catheter is threaded through a vein in the neck and guided into the liver. A biopsy needle is then advanced through the catheter to collect a sample. Transjugular biopsy is typically used when there is a risk of bleeding complications or when a percutaneous biopsy is not feasible.

Laparoscopic Liver Biopsy: This is a surgical procedure in which a laparoscope (a thin, flexible tube with a camera) is inserted through small incisions in the abdomen to view the liver. A tissue sample is collected using specialized instruments. Laparoscopic biopsy is less common but may be used when other methods are not suitable.

Liver biopsy is generally performed for the following reasons:

- To diagnose the cause of unexplained liver abnormalities, such as elevated liver enzymes or an enlarged liver.

- To assess the severity of liver diseases, such as hepatitis, cirrhosis, or fibrosis.
- To determine the extent of liver damage and guide treatment decisions.
- To evaluate liver tumors and distinguish between benign and malignant (cancerous) growths.

The procedure is usually done on an outpatient basis, and patients are often advised to avoid blood-thinning medications before the biopsy to reduce the risk of bleeding. After the biopsy, patients are typically observed for several hours to monitor for potential complications, such as bleeding or pain. Recovery time is usually short, and patients can resume normal activities within a few days.

Liver biopsy carries some risks, including bleeding and pain, but these risks are generally low when performed by experienced healthcare providers. The decision to undergo a liver biopsy is made based on the individual's medical history and the need for specific diagnostic information.

Chapter 13: Surgical Anatomy

Liver resection

Liver resection, also known as hepatectomy, is a surgical procedure to remove a portion of the liver. It is often performed to treat liver tumors, including both cancerous (malignant) and non-cancerous (benign) growths. Understanding the surgical anatomy of the liver is crucial for a successful liver resection. Here are some key aspects:

Liver Lobes: The liver is divided into two main lobes: the right lobe and the left lobe. The right lobe is larger and is further divided into the anterior (front) and posterior (back) segments. The left lobe is smaller and consists of the left lateral segment and the left medial segment.

Couinaud Classification: The Couinaud classification is a system used to describe the liver's anatomical segments. It divides the liver into eight functional segments based on blood supply and drainage. Each segment has its own vascular and biliary supply, making it possible to resect specific segments while preserving the remaining liver tissue.

Blood Supply: The liver has a dual blood supply. The hepatic artery brings oxygen-rich blood from the heart, while the portal vein carries nutrient-rich blood from the digestive organs. These blood vessels branch into smaller vessels within the liver.

Biliary System: The liver produces bile, which is essential for digestion. The bile ducts, including the common hepatic duct and common bile duct, transport bile to the gallbladder and small intestine. Understanding the biliary anatomy is important during liver resection to avoid damaging these ducts.

During a liver resection:

- The surgeon carefully identifies the blood vessels and bile ducts that supply the portion of the liver to be removed.
- The blood vessels are clamped and divided to control bleeding.
- The liver tissue is cut along specific anatomical planes to remove the targeted portion.

- After removal, the remaining liver tissue is carefully examined to ensure adequate blood flow and bile drainage.
- The cut edges of the liver may be sealed or sutured to prevent bleeding or bile leakage.
- The removed liver tissue is sent to a pathology lab for examination.

The goal of liver resection is to remove the diseased portion while preserving as much healthy liver tissue as possible to maintain liver function. The remaining liver can regenerate and compensate for the loss of tissue over time. However, not all patients are candidates for liver resection, and the decision depends on factors such as the location and size of the tumor, overall liver function, and the patient's overall health.

Liver resection is a complex surgical procedure that requires specialized training and expertise in hepatobiliary surgery. Patients undergoing liver resection are typically closely monitored before and after surgery to ensure a successful recovery.

Transplantation

A liver transplant is a surgical procedure in which a diseased or failing liver is replaced with a healthy liver from a deceased or living donor. Liver transplantation is considered when medical treatments and other interventions are no longer effective in treating end-stage liver disease or severe liver conditions. Here are key aspects of liver transplantation:

Indications for Liver Transplantation: Liver transplantation may be considered for various conditions, including:

- End-stage liver disease (cirrhosis) due to hepatitis B, hepatitis C, alcoholic liver disease, non-alcoholic fatty liver disease (NAFLD), autoimmune hepatitis, or other causes.
- Liver cancer (hepatocellular carcinoma) that meets specific criteria.
- Certain metabolic liver diseases.
- Acute liver failure caused by factors such as drug toxicity or viral infections.

Donor Types:

Deceased Donor: In most cases, the liver is obtained from a deceased donor who has been declared brain dead but has a viable liver. Deceased donor transplantation is the most common type.

Living Donor: In some situations, a portion of a healthy liver can be donated by a living individual, typically a family member or close friend. The remaining liver in both the donor and the recipient regenerates to near-normal size.

Transplant Surgery: The liver transplant surgery involves the removal of the diseased liver and its replacement with the healthy donor liver. The surgery can last several hours and requires specialized expertise.

Immunosuppression: After transplantation, recipients must take immunosuppressive medications for the rest of their lives to prevent their immune system from rejecting the new liver. Finding the right balance of immunosuppression is crucial to prevent rejection while avoiding complications.

Recovery and Rehabilitation: After surgery, recipients require a period of hospitalization and post-operative care. Recovery times vary but can be several weeks to months. Rehabilitation and ongoing medical follow-up are essential for a successful outcome.

Complications: Liver transplantation is a complex procedure and can be associated with various complications, including rejection of the transplanted liver, infection, side effects of immunosuppressive medications, and others. Close monitoring and prompt intervention are critical.

Long-Term Outcome: Liver transplantation can be life-saving and can greatly improve the quality of life for recipients. Many recipients can return to normal activities, but they require lifelong medical management and monitoring.

The success rate of liver transplantation has improved significantly over the years, thanks to advances in surgical techniques, immunosuppressive medications, and patient care. However, the availability of donor organs is limited, and transplant candidates are prioritized based on medical urgency. As a result, not all individuals with liver disease are suitable candidates for transplantation.

Liver transplantation is a complex medical procedure that requires a multidisciplinary team of healthcare professionals, including transplant surgeons, hepatologists, nurses, and others, to provide comprehensive care to recipients before, during, and after the transplant. The decision to undergo liver transplantation is made based on careful evaluation and consideration of the patient's medical condition and overall health.

Surgical considerations

Surgical considerations for liver procedures, including liver resection, transplantation, and other interventions, involve several important factors that surgeons must take into account to ensure successful outcomes. Here are some key surgical considerations related to liver surgery:

Patient Evaluation: Before any liver surgery, a thorough evaluation of the patient's medical history, liver function, overall health, and any underlying medical conditions is essential. This evaluation helps determine whether the patient is a suitable candidate for surgery and assesses the risks involved.

Liver Function: Evaluating the functional capacity of the liver is crucial. This often involves blood tests to assess liver enzymes, bilirubin levels, and clotting factors. A compromised liver function may affect the surgical approach and postoperative recovery.

Tumor Assessment: In cases of liver cancer, it's essential to assess the tumor's location, size, and extent within the liver. This information guides decisions about whether the tumor can be resected, the type of resection needed, or whether transplantation is a better option.

Imaging: Preoperative imaging, such as CT scans, MRI scans, or ultrasound, provides detailed information about the liver's anatomy, including the location of blood vessels and bile ducts. Surgeons use this imaging to plan the surgical approach and identify anatomical variations.

Vascular Control: Managing blood flow within the liver during surgery is critical to prevent excessive bleeding. Surgeons often use vascular occlusion techniques, like Pringle maneuver or selective clamping, to control blood flow to the liver during resection.

Biliary Anatomy: Understanding the biliary system's anatomy is crucial to avoid damaging bile ducts during surgery. Bile duct injuries can lead to significant complications, such as bile leaks.

Intraoperative Ultrasound: Surgeons may use intraoperative ultrasound to visualize the liver in real-time during surgery. This helps identify tumors, assess the extent of resection, and confirm that the planned resection margins are clear.

Minimally Invasive Techniques: In some cases, minimally invasive techniques, such as laparoscopic or robotic-assisted surgery, may be used for liver procedures. These approaches can result in smaller incisions, reduced pain, and quicker recovery times.

Liver Regeneration: Understanding the liver's regenerative capacity is important, especially in living donor liver transplantation, where a portion of the donor's liver is removed. The remaining liver tissue in both the donor and recipient must regenerate to near-normal size.

Postoperative Care: Appropriate postoperative care, including monitoring for complications such as bleeding, infection, or bile leaks, is crucial for patient recovery. Managing pain, nutrition, and immunosuppressive medications (in transplantation) are also essential.

Long-Term Follow-Up: Patients who undergo liver surgery require long-term follow-up to monitor for recurrence of liver conditions, assess liver function, and adjust treatment as needed.

Liver surgery is complex and demands precision, careful planning, and a multidisciplinary approach involving surgeons, hepatologists, anesthesiologists, radiologists, and other healthcare professionals. The choice of surgical technique and approach depends on the specific condition being treated and the patient's individual circumstances. Surgeons aim to balance effective treatment with minimizing risks and preserving liver function.

Chapter 14: Maintaining Liver Health

Healthy lifestyle choices

Maintaining a healthy lifestyle is crucial for supporting liver health and preventing liver disease. Here are some healthy lifestyle choices that can help promote liver health:

Balanced Diet: Eating a well-balanced diet can help prevent fatty liver disease and promote liver health. Focus on:

- A variety of fruits and vegetables for vitamins, antioxidants, and fiber.
- Lean sources of protein like poultry, fish, beans, and tofu.
- Whole grains for complex carbohydrates.
- Limiting saturated and trans fats, sugary foods, and excess salt.

Moderate Alcohol Consumption: If person choose to consume alcohol, do so in moderation. Excessive alcohol intake can lead to alcoholic liver disease, cirrhosis, and liver cancer. Guidelines vary, but moderate drinking typically means up to one drink per day for women and up to two drinks per day for men.

Stay Hydrated: Drinking plenty of water helps the liver perform its functions effectively. It also aids in digestion and detoxification.

Exercise Regularly: Engaging in regular physical activity helps control weight, reduce the risk of non-alcoholic fatty liver disease (NAFLD), and improve overall health.

Maintain a Healthy Weight: Obesity is a risk factor for NAFLD and can contribute to liver disease. Achieving and maintaining a healthy weight through diet and exercise is important.

Avoid Risky Behaviors: Protect from hepatitis infections by practicing safe sex, avoiding sharing needles or personal items that may be contaminated, and getting vaccinated for hepatitis A and B if recommended.

Medication Management: Be cautious with medications and supplements. Some medications, including over-the-counter drugs and herbal supplements, can be harmful to the liver. Always follow dosage instructions.

Vaccination: Consider getting vaccinated for hepatitis A and B if they at risk or if healthcare provider recommends it. These vaccines can prevent these viral infections, which can lead to liver damage.

Limit Exposure to Toxins: Be mindful of exposure to chemicals and toxins at home and work. Properly handle and store household chemicals, and follow safety guidelines at workplace if they work with potentially harmful substances.

Practice Safe Tattooing and Piercing: Ensure that any equipment used for tattoos or body piercings is properly sterilized to reduce the risk of infection with hepatitis B or C.

Regular Health Check-Ups: Attend regular check-ups with healthcare provider. Routine blood tests can help detect liver problems early when they are often more treatable.

Manage Chronic Conditions: If person have chronic conditions like diabetes or high blood pressure, manage them effectively, as they can impact liver health.

Reduce Stress: High levels of stress can affect their overall health, including liver health. Incorporate stress-reduction techniques like meditation, yoga, or deep breathing into daily routine.

Adopting these healthy lifestyle choices can significantly reduce the risk of liver disease and support overall well-being. If patient have concerns about liver health or are at risk due to family history or other factors, it's important to discuss them with a healthcare provider for personalized guidance and monitoring.

Diet and nutrition

Maintaining liver health through diet and nutrition is crucial, as a healthy diet can help prevent liver disease and support overall liver function. Here are dietary guidelines for promoting liver health:

Consume a Well-Balanced Diet: A balanced diet provides essential nutrients that support liver function. Include a variety of foods, such as:

- **Fruits and vegetables:** Rich in vitamins, antioxidants, and fiber.
- **Lean protein sources:** Choose lean meats, poultry, fish, tofu, beans, and legumes.
- **Whole grains:** Opt for whole-grain bread, pasta, rice, and cereals for complex carbohydrates.
- **Healthy fats:** Include sources like avocados, nuts, seeds, and olive oil.
- **Dairy or dairy alternatives:** Incorporate low-fat or fat-free dairy products or plant-based alternatives.

Limit Saturated and Trans Fats: High intake of saturated and trans fats can contribute to fatty liver disease. Reduce consumption of fried foods, processed snacks, and fatty cuts of meat.

Reduce Sugar and Sugary Beverages: Excessive sugar intake can lead to non-alcoholic fatty liver disease (NAFLD). Minimize consumption of sugary drinks, sweets, and foods with added sugars.

Moderate Alcohol Consumption: Limit alcohol consumption or avoid it altogether, as excessive alcohol can harm the liver and lead to alcoholic liver disease. If choose to drink, do so in moderation.

Control Portion Sizes: Pay attention to portion sizes to avoid overeating and excessive calorie intake, which can contribute to obesity and fatty liver disease.

Stay Hydrated: Drinking enough water supports overall health, including liver function. Aim for an adequate daily intake of fluids.

Choose Lean Proteins: Opt for lean sources of protein, such as skinless poultry, fish, tofu, legumes, and low-fat dairy products. Reducing red meat consumption may be beneficial.

Limit Salt Intake: High salt intake can lead to fluid retention and contribute to liver problems. Reduce your consumption of high-sodium foods, including processed and fast foods.

Include Fiber-Rich Foods: High-fiber foods, such as whole grains, fruits, vegetables, and legumes, can aid digestion and promote a healthy gut, indirectly benefiting the liver.

Consider Antioxidant-Rich Foods: Antioxidants found in fruits and vegetables help protect liver cells from damage caused by free radicals. Berries, citrus fruits, and leafy greens are excellent choices.

Moderate Caffeine Intake: Some studies suggest that moderate caffeine consumption may have protective effects on the liver. Coffee and tea are sources of caffeine, but excessive caffeine intake should be avoided.

Limit Processed Foods: Processed foods often contain additives, preservatives, and unhealthy fats that can negatively affect liver health. Focus on whole, unprocessed foods.

Maintain a Healthy Weight: If overweight or obese, aim for gradual weight loss through a combination of a balanced diet and regular exercise to reduce the risk of fatty liver disease.

Consider Dietary Supplements Carefully: Talk to a healthcare provider before taking dietary supplements or herbal remedies, as some can be harmful to the liver.

Remember that individual dietary needs can vary, especially if they have liver disease or specific dietary concerns.

Liver detoxification myths

Liver detoxification myths are common misconceptions about how the liver functions and how certain diets or products can cleanse or detoxify the liver. It's important to debunk these myths and rely on accurate information about liver health. Here are some common liver detoxification myths:

Myth: Need a Detox Diet to Cleanse Liver: The liver is a highly efficient organ that naturally detoxifies the body by processing and eliminating toxins. There is no need for special detox diets or products to "cleanse" the liver. Eating a balanced diet and maintaining a healthy lifestyle is sufficient for liver health.

Myth: Juice Cleanses and Detox Teas Improve Liver Function: Many commercial juice cleanses and detox teas claim to remove toxins from the liver. However, these products often lack scientific evidence to support their effectiveness. A well-balanced diet provides the nutrients the liver needs to function optimally.

Myth: Liver Flushes or Gallbladder Flushes Remove Gallstones: Liver or gallbladder flushes involve consuming specific mixtures of oil and juice to flush out gallstones. These procedures are not medically proven and can be risky. Genuine gallstones are typically not expelled through these methods.

Myth: Fasting or Extreme Calorie Restriction Helps Liver Detoxification: Extreme fasting or calorie restriction can lead to nutrient deficiencies and harm liver health. The liver requires a consistent supply of nutrients to function properly. Crash diets can stress the liver and lead to muscle loss.

Myth: Certain Foods or Supplements Purge Toxins from the Liver: While some foods, like cruciferous vegetables, contain compounds that support liver health, they do not act as miracle detoxifiers. Consuming a variety of nutritious foods is more effective than relying on a single "superfood."

Myth: Should Feel Physical Symptoms During a Liver Detox: Some detox programs claim that should experience symptoms like headaches, fatigue, or skin rashes as evidence that toxins are leaving your body. In reality, these symptoms can be signs of dehydration, nutrient deficiencies, or the side effects of extreme diets.

Myth: Liver Detox Diets Cure Chronic Liver Diseases: Detox diets cannot cure chronic liver diseases like cirrhosis, hepatitis, or fatty liver disease.

These conditions often require medical management and lifestyle changes.

Myth: Liver Cleanses Can Prevent Liver Cancer: While maintaining liver health is important for overall well-being, liver cleanses or detox diets do not provide protection against liver cancer. Reducing risk factors like excessive alcohol consumption and hepatitis infection is more important.

Myth: It Can Overload the Liver with Toxins: The liver has a remarkable capacity to handle toxins. It is not easily overwhelmed by everyday exposures. Chronic, excessive alcohol consumption, drug abuse, or exposure to toxic substances over a long period can harm the liver.

It's essential to base decisions about liver health on reliable medical advice and scientific evidence.

Summary

The liver is a vital organ in the human body with complex anatomy and functions. Here is a summary of the key aspects of liver anatomy:

Location: The liver is located in the upper right abdomen, just below the diaphragm and under the ribcage.

Size: It is the largest internal organ, weighing about 3 pounds (1.4 kilograms) in adults.

Lobes: The liver is divided into two main lobes: the right lobe and the left lobe. The right lobe is larger, while the left lobe is smaller.

Segments: The liver is further divided into eight functional segments based on blood supply and drainage, as defined by the Couinaud classification.

Blood Supply: Blood enters the liver through two main vessels: the hepatic artery, which carries oxygenated blood from the heart, and the portal vein, which carries nutrient-rich blood from the digestive organs. These blood vessels branch into smaller vessels within the liver.

Biliary System: The liver produces bile, a digestive fluid. Bile is transported through a network of bile ducts, including the common hepatic duct and common bile duct, which eventually connect to the gallbladder and small intestine.

Functions:

- **Metabolism:** The liver plays a central role in metabolizing carbohydrates, fats, and proteins.
- **Detoxification:** It detoxifies harmful substances, including drugs and toxins, from the bloodstream.
- **Synthesis:** The liver synthesizes proteins, including albumin and clotting factors.
- **Storage:** It stores glycogen (for energy), vitamins, and minerals.
- **Blood Filtration:** The liver filters and cleanses the blood of impurities.

Regeneration: The liver has remarkable regenerative capabilities. It can regrow lost tissue and return to near-normal function even after partial removal.

Surrounding Structures: The liver is closely connected to other abdominal organs, including the gallbladder, pancreas, and intestines.

Understanding liver anatomy is essential for diagnosing and treating liver conditions, as well as for performing surgical procedures like liver resection and transplantation. The liver's complexity and its role in various metabolic and physiological processes make it a crucial organ for maintaining overall health.

Liver anatomy is a complex and specialized field of study, and there are several textbooks that provide comprehensive information on the topic. Here is a reference to a well-regarded book on liver anatomy:

Book Title: "Anatomy of the Liver, Gallbladder, and Biliary System: The Sectional Atlas of MRI and CT"

Author: Dr. Suriya prakash R

Publisher: Suriya prakash

Publication Year: 2023

1st edition

This book focuses on the anatomy of the liver, gallbladder, and biliary system, with a specific emphasis on using MRI and CT imaging techniques to visualize and understand the anatomy. It includes detailed illustrations, images, and sectional views that aid in the study of liver anatomy.

Please note that the field of medical textbooks is constantly evolving, and there may be newer editions or alternative textbooks available that also cover liver anatomy in detail. You may want to consult with your educational institution or a medical library for the most up-to-date resources on this topic.